ASK DR. WEIL

COMMON ILLNESSES

By Andrew Weil, M.D.:

Ask Dr. Weil
WOMEN'S HEALTH
YOUR TOP HEALTH CONCERNS
NATURAL REMEDIES
VITAMINS AND MINERALS
COMMON ILLNESSES
HEALTHY LIVING

8 WEEKS TO OPTIMUM HEALTH
SPONTANEOUS HEALING
NATURAL HEALTH, NATURAL MEDICINE
HEALTH AND HEALING
FROM CHOCOLATE TO MORPHINE
THE MARRIAGE OF THE SUN AND THE MOON
THE NATURAL MIND

ASK DR. WEIL

COMMON ILLNESSES

Andrew Weil, M.D.

Edited by Steven Petrow

IVY BOOKS • NEW YORK

All material provided in the Ask Dr. Weil program is provided for educational purposes only. Consult your own physician regarding the applicability of any opinions or recommendations with respect to your symptoms or medical condition.

Questions contained in this book may appear in other volumes of the Ask Dr. Weil series. The books are arranged according to topic, and to create a complete health profile utilizing Dr. Weil's prescriptions, material may overlap.

Ivy Books
Published by Ballantine Books
 Published in the United States by Ballantine Books, a division of Random House, Inc., New York, and simultaneously in Canada by Random House of Canada Limited, Toronto. This work was compiled from the "Ask Dr. Weil" Web site.

ISBN 0-8041-1676-8

Manufactured in the United States of America

Introduction

You've taken the first step toward optimum health. This book will give you more information about my philosophy along with answers to some of the questions I am asked most frequently.

I wrote *Spontaneous Healing* and *8 Weeks to Optimum Health* because I wanted to call attention to the innate, intrinsic nature of the healing process. I've always believed that the body can heal itself if you give it a chance. Why? Because it has a healing system. If you're feeling well, it's important to know about this system so that you can enhance your well-being. If you are ill, you'll also want to know about it because it is your best hope of recovery.

To maintain optimum health requires commitment. This book—and the others in the series—can give you much of the basic information you need about diet, supplements, common illnesses, natural remedies, and healthy living.

All of these questions originated on "Ask Dr. Weil," my program on the World Wide Web. If you still have questions, come visit the clinic at www.drweil.com.

How to Fight Athlete's Foot?

Q:

My feet are itchy. Is grapefruit seed extract really as good for athlete's foot as the guy at the health food store claims?

A:

Athlete's foot is a fungal infection of the skin, related to jock itch and ringworm. As you probably know, it thrives in moist, warm, dark places, so one of the best treatments I can recommend is exposing your feet to fresh air and sunlight. Keep them clean and dry—and wear sandals if you can.

I've also heard a lot of positive testimonials about grapefruit seed extract, which is available at health food stores. It is reported to have significant antifungal effects. Apply the extract (full strength) two to three times a day to the affected area.

Tea tree oil, extracted from the leaves of *Melaleuca alternifolia*, a tree native to Australia, is another home remedy that works as well as or better than over-the-counter medications like Tinactin and Lotrimin. Apply a light coating of the oil to the affected area three or four times a day, and continue to apply it for two weeks after the infection seems to have disappeared. You want to make sure the fungus is eradicated. Tea tree oil will also clear up fungal infections of the toenails or fingernails, conditions that are usually difficult to cure, even with strong systemic antibiotics. It's also effective for ringworm and jock itch as well as bacterial infections of the skin. You'll find tea tree oil products at health food and herb stores. Be sure to select ones that are 100 percent tea tree oil.

Plagued by an Aching Back?

Q:

What do I do for lower back pain?

A:

Chronic back pain is often caused by unbalanced nervous control of the musculature, which triggers muscle contraction, reduction of normal blood supply, and inflammation. In most cases, it's not directly caused by structural injury, although injury can create a focal point for the effects of neuromuscular imbalance.

What you're feeling is the end result of a chain of nervous system events that starts in your brain and leads to pain in your back. Because the nervous system is connected to the mind and the emotions, healing is best directed there, often the root of the trouble. This isn't to say that your pain is all in your head, but rather that the vicious cycle of muscle spasm may have an emotional root. John Sarno, M.D., calls most cases of chronic back pain "tension myositis syndrome," referring to psychosomatic inflammation of the muscles. He has a great book on the subject called *Healing Back Pain.*

So rather than looking to chiropractors, osteopaths, acupuncturists, or massage practitioners to cure the pain, I'd try to understand the real nature of the problem and consider mental and emotional changes. Sometimes it may do the trick just to understand that the pain can depart once your brain stops sending the wrong messages to your back. Think about restructuring the patterns of thinking, feeling, and managing stress that lead your nervous system to spasm.

You can take steps to strengthen your back and improve the health of the muscles that contribute to the pain. Yoga is a wonderful way to improve flexibility and balance your nervous system. Stretches that target your hamstrings are a good way to make sure your back gets the support it needs. Abdominal strengthening exercises will also help.

The way you sit is important, too, especially if you spend long days at a computer or a desk. Sit a bit forward on your chair, with your knees comfortably apart and heels on the floor, your pelvis rotated slightly forward with your body balanced on top. If you place a rolled-up towel under your tailbone, it will help you achieve a good sitting posture. Don't puff out your chest; that's hard on your back, too.

There may also be a link between back pain and diet. One study found that arteries narrowed by atherosclerosis—avoidable with a low-fat diet—can't deliver as much blood to the lower back, and this affects disks, muscles, and nerves.

If you have an episode of acute lower back pain, use ice on the area as soon as you can. Chiropractic manipulation has also been shown to help. And keep in mind that almost everyone who suffers from acute back pain recovers in about a month with or without treatment.

Black-Eye Blues?

Q:

About three days ago I received a black eye while playing football. The swelling is down, but what is the best thing I can do to get the discoloration out of my eye? Is there any type of lotion that will speed up the healing process and remove the black and purple ring?

A:

A black eye is just a big bruise that happens to be in a very noticeable place. The first thing to do—which it sounds as if you've already done—is put cold on it. Immediately. That keeps the swelling down and may reduce the amount of bruising.

It is possible to speed up the healing process by taking the pineapple enzyme bromelain. You can buy bromelain in capsule form in health food stores. It is absorbed through the digestive tract and promotes healing of tissue injuries. Take 200 to 400 milligrams three times a day on an empty stomach (not within two hours of eating). A few individuals have allergic reactions to bromelain; discontinue if you get any itching.

Homeopathic arnica would also probably be a good idea, because it helps the body recover faster from trauma. Buy *Arnica montana* in 30x potency at a health food store, and let the tablets dissolve under your tongue. (Do not handle them. Shake them into the bottle cap and then toss them in your mouth.) Take four tablets immediately, then four every hour while awake the first day. The second day, cut back to four tablets every two hours; then four tablets four times a day. Continue the treatment four to five days. You may also want to rub some arnica tincture on the bruise, making sure to keep the arnica out of the eye itself.

In the meantime, keep smiling, and come up with a really enthralling story about your football adventure. You might also wear sunglasses!

Blood in My Stool?

Q:

My boyfriend has just told me that he noticed blood in his stool and in the toilet after having a bowel movement. He is afraid to call the doctor and insists he'll wait and see if it happens again. I'm worried, though. What could this be symptomatic of?

A:

You're wise to pay attention. But your boyfriend may be right about waiting until it happens again. If he's in his twenties or thirties, the cause could be a number of things—none of them likely to be terribly serious. Hemorrhoids and ulcers can put blood in your stool. An inflammatory condition called diverticulitis in the colon could also be the cause.

In younger people, the most common reason for blood in the stool is a hemorrhoid or fissure very near the anus. There is also the possibility—if there is also pain—that the cause is inflamed rectal tissue from a sexually transmitted disease such as gonorrhea or herpes. In general, bright red blood is coming from a site close to the anus. Blood from higher up in the digestive tract, such as from a bleeding ulcer, will look black and tarry. Small amounts of blood leaking into the gastrointestinal tract can be invisible or "occult." Doctors use a simple color test to reveal occult blood in a tiny amount of stool obtained from a rectal examination, and this should be done as part of every physical exam.

Older people should be very alert to blood in the stool because it can be a sign of colon cancer and always should be investigated. Colon cancer is curable only in its early stages, so it's very important to catch it right away. In this case it would be prudent to have a sigmoidoscopy. A sigmoidoscope is a long tube with a light at the end, which allows your doctor to get a direct look at the lining of the colon just above the anus, where most cancers arise. It can reveal polyps—mushroom-shaped growths that can be precancerous—as well as early malignant growths. There's also colonoscopy, a similar but more elaborate procedure to examine the entire colon with a fiberoptic scope. Other signs of colon cancer that might accompany blood in the stool are changes in bowel habits and in shape or consistency of stools.

Lower Your Risk for Breast Cancer?

Q:

What specific things can women do to reduce the risk of breast cancer? It's well-publicized that early breast-feeding is helpful. Can you give specific dietary recommendations or other suggestions? Thanks.

A:

Breast cancer results from a complex interaction of genetic and environmental factors. While we do not know all the details of its origin, we can make specific recommendations for lifestyle changes that will reduce risk. Some of these are intended to reduce estrogen production in the body or limit exposure to foreign estrogens. Those hormones stimulate breast cells to grow and divide, increasing the chance of malignant transformation. Other recommendations are aimed at strengthening the body's defenses.

Women who begin menstruating early have a higher risk of breast cancer, as do those who reach menopause late. Such women are exposed to estrogen for longer periods of time. Having a first baby at a younger age and breast-feeding both lessen the risk of breast cancer, probably by interrupting the menstrual cycle and reducing lifetime estrogen exposure. You may not be able to change much here, but you can make choices about your diet that will affect the amount of estrogen in your body.

Animal fats contribute to increased estrogen levels in the body, and a low-fat diet has been shown to help guard against breast cancer. Commercially raised animal foods often contain residues of estrogenic hormones given to animals as growth promoters. If you are a carnivore, you should check out Laura's Lean Beef at (800) ITS LEAN (487-5326). Laura Freeman runs a family farm outside Winchester, Kentucky, and all the beef is hormone- and antibiotic-free.

Soy products such as tofu, tempeh, and miso, which are full of weak, plant-based estrogens, lower cancer risk, perhaps because they occupy estrogen receptors, protecting them from stronger forms of the hormone (including many environmental pollutants). Compounds in cabbage block stronger surges of estrogen from other sources. Compounds in broccoli, kale, and collard greens also may be helpful.

On the other hand, alcohol, even in moderate usage, can increase estrogen production in susceptible women.

Regular, moderate exercise—four hours a week—reduced breast cancer risk before menopause by an average of 58 percent in one study. Researchers believe it lowers estrogen production. After menopause, exercise may still help by lessening body fat, another factor in estrogen exposure.

So the most important thing to think about is protecting the overall health and well-being of your body. Exercise regularly. Minimize your exposure to environmental estrogenic pollutants by eating low on the food chain. Especially limit your intake of commercially raised meats, dairy products, and eggs. Eat lots of organic fruits, vegetables, and soy foods and plenty of fiber to keep estrogen levels under control and protect your genes from damage. Also, take antioxidants to guard against deleterious mutations and protect immune defenses.

If you know you're at high risk, take two tablespoons of ground flaxseed on your cereal or in your juice every day. Flaxseed reduces the rate of growth of tumors in rats and lowers the chance of cancer's getting started in the first place.

Finally, note that the role of psychological factors in breast cancer is not at all clear. Grief and depression may suppress immunity, allowing cancers to grow faster. But I doubt that they play much of a role in their origin. Women with this disease did not "give themselves cancer" as a result of any sort of emotional failure.

Looking for Alternatives in Cancer Care?

Q:

Do you know of a reputable center for alternative cancer therapy?

A:

There is no one right treatment for cancer. And, unfortunately, there is no one magical alternative out there.

First, I'd determine just what sort of help is needed. Michael Lerner has written an excellent book, *Choice in Healing,* on integrating alternative and conventional treatments. As Lerner recommends, it's important to consider three factors: the plausibility of the therapy itself, the character of the practitioner, and the quality of service at the center. I would ask you to also consider the expense and practicality of going to any treatment center. An appendix in Lerner's book describes specific therapies and their better-known practitioners.

For cancers that are growing rapidly, the benefits of chemotherapy or radiation may outweigh the risks. If you decide to use the conventional therapies, then I would look for guidance on nutrition, dietary supplements, and mind-body techniques all of which can increase their effectiveness and reduce their toxicity. Many of the alternative cancer centers use this approach.

If you decide not to use conventional therapies, then you'll need to shop around and evaluate success rates of other treatments. Some centers use therapies that are not accepted by the medical establishment, even though the centers may be staffed by M.D.s. I don't know that there's any one approach that has consistent success, although there are well-documented cases of individuals who have done well on alternative regimens.

Interesting practitioners include Dr. Nicholas Gonzalez in New York City and Dr. Stanislaw Burzynski in Houston, Texas, both of whom are M.D.s. Dr. Gonzalez is using an updated version of a complex nutritional therapy developed by the late William D. Kelley, a dentist from Texas. The treatment involves highly individualized diets; massive vitamin, mineral, and enzyme supplementation, and detoxification using coffee enemas. Dr. Burzynski focuses his work on antineoplastons, peptide molecules he discovered in human urine. There is considerable controversy over the effectiveness of his very expensive therapy. In fact, a recent case in federal court (brought by the government) sought to determine whether Burzynski was guilty of violating federal regulations in his use of an unapproved cancer treatment. It ended in a hung jury.

Treatments at many alternative cancer clinics are expensive, and, of course, insurance doesn't cover them. It's a good idea to see if the place you're considering will put you in touch with people who have been there. If they won't do that, I would be suspicious. Consider especially what sort of success the practitioner may have had with the specific type of cancer you're dealing with. I'd also talk to other cancer specialists, and to nurses and other medical assistants who work in the clinic.

Crippled by Carpal Tunnel Syndrome?

Q:

Due to repetitive typing I have developed carpal tunnel syndrome in both arms. I was given anti-inflammatory medication for this. Then I developed stomach problems—gastritis and irritable bowel syndrome. After two years of getting all kinds of tests done and having doctors tell me that I was going to have to live with this the rest of my life, I got fed up. What do you recommend?

A:

When you're an especially speedy typist or spend long hours at the keyboard, the tendons that move the fingers can swell. There's one little tunnel of ligamentous tissue at the base of your palm that all the tendons and one very important nerve pass through from your arm to your hand. That's where the swelling and pressure can become especially painful and irritating, causing a condition known as carpal tunnel syndrome (CTS).

The most effective treatment that I've found is vitamin

B-6 (pyridoxine), 100 milligrams, two or three times a day. In this dosage, pyridoxine is not acting as a B vitamin but rather as a natural therapeutic agent that relieves nerve compression injuries. Be aware that doses of B-6 higher than 300 milligrams a day have caused rare cases of nerve damage. Discontinue usage if you develop any unusual numbness. (A much-publicized University of Michigan study warned about nerve toxicity with B-6 and discouraged people from using it for CTS. I disagree.)

For quick relief when you're hurting, rub on arnica gel, which you can find in your health food store or drugstore. Also, try wrapping ice packs around your wrists (a bag of frozen peas works just as well); if you use this treatment for five minutes every few hours when you're especially stressing your wrists, it may ease the pain and the inflammation. Ginger tablets with DYL (deglycyrrhizinated licorice) may relieve inflammation, and acupuncture certainly can provide symptomatic relief.

The most important consideration when you've got CTS is to figure out ways to reduce your typing. Unless you reduce the strain on your wrists, long-term improvement is unlikely. That means less typing, and learning how to stop driving yourself so hard at the keyboard.

There are a couple of other things you can try. Make yourself stand up every hour for a few minutes and stretch. The muscles in your wrists are connected all the way up through your arms, across your shoulders, and up into your neck. Pay attention to those parts of your body, too, because stretching and relaxing your shoulders, neck, and back can ease the strain on your wrists. I know some people who've found a lot of relief through deep-tissue massage or Rolfing. And consider whether you're feeling some emotional tension at work that tightens your whole body, making it more susceptible to injury.

Your posture at the keyboard can make a big difference. Sit up straight, with your weight slightly forward. Your feet should be flat on the floor, or tilted comfortably on an adjustable footrest. An adjustable keyboard tray allows you to change the position of your hands now and then, and helps you keep your wrists straight, with your forearms horizontal and at a 90-degree angle to your upper arms. Your elbows should be at your sides in a relaxed position. Every now and then, tilt your head slowly to each side, and roll your shoulders twice forward and twice back. Squeeze your hands into tight fists and then stretch your fingers out as wide as they will go. Close your hands into fists again and rotate your wrists a few times in either direction.

You can also try a different keyboard. Each brand has its own key touch and key width, some of which may feel better to you than others. If you can find a split keyboard, it may help you to keep your hands and arms at a more natural angle. There are also some new keyboards with concave keys, sections tilted up like an accordion, and other unusual shapes. I haven't tried them, but you may want to check them out.

Caught a Cold?

Q:

I've spent too much money on all those fancy over-the-counter products for colds. Sometimes they mask the symptoms, but they don't really seem to make me better. Any other recommendations?

A:

You're absolutely right. Most of the over-the-counter products don't help you heal, even if they do stop the sniffles and headaches for a short while. I learned recently that more over-the-counter products are sold for the common cold than for any other disease. Not really surprising. Over the years, I have been collecting home remedies for colds—using myself and my family as guinea pigs. Here's what I've found works best:

Take vitamin C to prevent colds—1,000 to 2,000 milligrams, three times a day. Start this now if you get more than two colds a year.

As soon as you start feeling cold symptoms, eat two

cloves (not heads) of raw garlic. Trust me on this. You may not be kissing anyone soon, but garlic has powerful antibiotic effects. Chop it up and mix it with food, or swallow larger pieces like pills.

You can also take echinacea (*Echinacea purpurea* and related species) at the first sign of a cold or flu—like a scratchy throat or achy back. Take a dropperful of the tincture in a little warm water (or tea) four times a day. Use half doses for children.

Try sucking on zinc gluconate or zinc acetate lozenges, which, according to a recent study, may cut the duration of a cold in half.

Finally, drink this powerful gingerroot tea for head and chest congestion, malaise, and the chills. Here's my recipe:

> Grate a 1-inch piece of peeled gingerroot. Put it in a pot with 2 cups of cold water, bring to a boil, lower heat, and simmer five minutes. Add 1/2 teaspoon cayenne pepper (or more or less to taste) and simmer one minute more. Remove from heat. Add 2 tablespoons of fresh lemon juice, honey to taste, and 1 or 2 cloves of mashed garlic. Let cool slightly, and strain if you desire.

Then get under the covers and drink as much of it as you like. Hope you feel better.

Going Crazy with Crabs?

Q:

Could crab lice be transmitted in the steam room of a gym? I assure you, I have not had sexual activity for the past six months. Somehow, I got crabs and I am embarrassed to go to my doctor. He probably won't believe me.

A:

First of all, never let embarrassment stop you from going to a doctor. It's part of his or her job not to make judgments, and besides, doctors have seen it all. I know! If your doctor makes you feel ashamed, then you're going to the wrong doctor.

Sexual contact is the most common method of transmitting crabs, but there are plenty of other modes. You can get crabs from sharing the clothing, bedding, or towels of an infested person. However, the temperature in the steam room would make it difficult for the lice to survive and hop from one person to another, so, frankly, I think you must have gotten them from another source.

Many years ago, a friend of mine told me that he once had a houseguest who shared towels with everyone in the house (a married couple and their three teenage children included). Unfortunately, the guest had crabs, and soon, so did everyone else in the house. Very quietly a "health emergency" was proclaimed, treatment and cleaning were begun, and the houseguest was sent away. I wonder what Miss Manners would have to say about that!

Crab lice get their name because they look very much like miniature crabs. Once on the body, they cling between two hairs, bury their heads underneath the skin, and feed on blood. They attach their tiny white eggs to hairs. The biting and moving around makes for severe itching and irritation. It doesn't take very many crabs to cause great discomfort. And they multiply very quickly.

You can get rid of crab lice just as you would head lice. One popular preparation is Kwell, which is 1 percent lindane, but it's toxic to people as well as lice. Lindane, a cousin of DDT, is easily absorbed into the skin and can affect the central nervous system. You're better off using one of the newer and safer products. Pyrethrum is a natural insecticide from a chrysanthemum relative. Neem, made from a tree in India, is another natural alternative. You can find them in garden stores.

Or use a treatment recommended by Kathi Keville in *Herbs for Health and Healing*, adapted for the pubic area:

2 ounces vegetable oil
20 drops tea tree essential oil
10 drops each, essential oils of rosemary, lavender, and lemon

Combine ingredients and first test them on the inside of your elbow for several hours. If there is no sign of irritation, then apply the treatment to your dry pubic hair. Cover the area with plastic wrap, followed by a towel. Leave these coverings on for one hour. Then work shampoo into the hair to cut the oil, rinse, and shampoo and rinse again. You'll probably need to do this a week later to get rid of any newly hatched lice.

And don't forget to clean all your towels, bed linens, and infested clothing. You don't want to become reinfested.

Cursing Your Cramps?

Q:

Is there any other way to stop cramps while having my period—other than with painkillers?

A:

Two-thirds of all women suffer from menstrual cramps. Until a couple of decades ago, the pain they endured was written off as a psychological "female problem" that women created for themselves. But in the late 1970s, researchers discovered a hormone called prostaglandin F_2 alpha that is released as the uterine lining breaks down, causing the uterus to go into spasm and hurt.

You can moderate the release of PGF_2 alpha through some dietary measures, primarily a low-fat, high–complex carbohydrate diet. Don't eat dairy products, and ease up on the meat and eggs. Cut back on fried foods and commercially baked foods. Most important, make sure you get enough essential fatty acids. If you have plenty of essential fatty acids in your system, your body will produce less

PGF_2 alpha and more of a different hormone that helps prevent cramps. In one study, women who took 1.8 grams of omega-3 fatty acids in fish-oil capsules twice a day for two months had a significant improvement in cramps, nausea, and headaches. They used half as much aspirin as they had previously. I know other women who say oil of evening primrose works wonderfully for the same pupose, at a dose of two to three 500-milligram capsules twice a day.

In *Women's Bodies, Women's Wisdom*, Christiane Northrup, M.D., recommends a series of supplements to protect against cramps: 100 milligrams of vitamin B-6 per day, 50 IU of vitamin E (in the form of d-alpha-tocopherol) three times a day, and 100 milligrams of magnesium three to four times a day. While you're menstruating, she suggests 100 milligrams of magnesium every two hours to ease pain.

There are some effective traditional remedies for cramps as well, such as raspberry leaf tea. It's nontoxic, so you can consume as much as you like. An herb called cramp bark (*Viburnum opulus*), from a European bush, is a stronger remedy. The dose is one dropperful of the tincture in warm water as needed.

I'd also try acupuncture. There are pressure points that some people say will help, such as the acupuncture point on the wrist that's used for alleviating nausea, or a point on the inside of the foot that's used by reflexologists.

Smoking has been linked to added menstrual pain. And remember how much of an influence stress can be. Try to reduce stress in your life and practice relaxation techniques, such as meditation or yoga.

Fight Depression Without Drugs?

Q:

What alternatives are there to conventional antidepressant medications or EST (electroshock therapy)? I have tried every medical therapy possible—except EST—but still face recurrent spontaneous episodes of major depression. Are there any alternative treatments that might halt this escalating cycle?

A:

There are only two alternative treatments for depression that I have any confidence in. The first is regular aerobic exercise, which can definitely provide a long-term solution. You'll have to do at least thirty minutes of some vigorous aerobic activity at least five times a week, and be prepared to wait several weeks before you see any benefit. Aerobic exercise is a preventive as well as a treatment.

The second is an herbal treatment, called Saint-John's-wort (*Hypericum perforatum*). Saint-John's-wort is much used in Germany for the treatment of mild to moderate depression, as well as associated disturbed sleep cycles. Take 300 milligrams three times a day, of a standardized extract containing at least 0.125 percent hypericin. Again, be prepared to wait two months before you see the full benefit.

Changes in your diet may also make a difference. Try eating less protein and fat, and more starches, fruits, and vegetables. Experiment with the following amino acid and vitamin formula, for which you can find all the ingredients in a health food store. First thing in the morning, take 1,500 milligrams of DL-phenylalanine (DLPA, an amino acid), 100 milligrams of vitamin B-6, and 500 milligrams of vitamin C, along with a piece of fruit or a small glass of juice. Don't eat again for at least an hour. (DLPA can worsen high blood pressure, so use the formula cautiously if you have this condition, and start with a dose of 100 milligrams while monitoring your blood pressure.) Take another 100 milligrams of B-6 and more vitamin C in the evening.

You say you've taken a variety of drugs for depression. In general, I think that the new generation of antidepressants, including Prozac, Zoloft, and Paxil, are less toxic and more effective than medications of the past. Collectively known as SSRIs, or selective serotonin-reuptake inhibitors, they interact with the regulating mechanism for the neurotransmitter serotonin in your brain. It's best to be cautious with any of these drugs, particularly because their makers would have you believe that no one can live a normal life without them.

Make sure you aren't taking any other medications that may contribute to depression. These include antihistamines, tranquilizers, sleeping pills, and narcotics. Recreational drugs, alcohol, and coffee can also make depression worse.

You make reference to EST—electroshock or electroconvulsive therapy. That is a last resort for the treatment of severe depression. It does work, but I hope things won't get to the point where that's your only option.

Psychiatrists tend to look at all mental problems as stemming from disordered brain chemistry; hence their emphasis on drugs. I believe that disordered moods could just as easily lead to biochemical changes in the brain, so I look elsewhere for treatments. Buddhist psychology views depression as the necessary consequence of seeking stimulation. It counsels us to cultivate emotional balance in life, rather than always seeking highs and then regretting the lows that follow. The prescription is daily meditation, and I agree this may be the best way to get at the root of depression and change it.

Truth About Endometriosis?

Q:

What special recommendations would you make regarding diet for endometriosis sufferers? Do you think this is an autoimmune disease?

A:

I don't know what the root cause of endometriosis is. Nobody does. It's a poorly understood disease, and the treatments are only partly helpful. The symptoms can be debilitating or just very bothersome: severe cramping, painful menstruation, intestinal problems, and sometimes depression. The condition is characterized by tissue that looks and behaves just like the lining of the uterus (endometrium), but grows elsewhere in the body: the abdominal cavity, the intestines, the ovaries, or the abdominal wall. And just like the lining of the uterus, this tissue builds up with hormonal changes over the month, then breaks down and bleeds. Blood in the abdomen causes intense inflammation that can be very painful. In some women, the result is severe scarring and organ dysfunction. Endometriosis is often associated with infertility, but hasn't been shown to cause it directly.

Endometriosis doesn't necessarily progress to damage within the pelvis, or contribute to infertility. Sometimes it's very hard to find it in the body, and more and more, doctors are learning that it's quite common, with as many as half of menstruating women living with it. So experts now believe that mild endometriosis may actually be normal, and not need any treatment. In fact, studies have found that in many instances it doesn't spread and grow worse over time at all.

The most popular theory about endometriosis rests on the idea that menstrual flow sometimes moves backwards and up through the fallopian tubes, then out into areas within the pelvis. There, the discarded tissue seems to implant and begin to grow. The hypothesis you mention is one of the most recent—that the immune system is misbehaving, failing to kill off stray endometrial cells and then pumping up their growth. Women with painful endometriosis often make antibodies against their own tissue, the hallmark of autoimmunity.

It's commonly held that pregnancy will protect against endometriosis, but recent studies have found no difference in incidence between women who have been pregnant and those who have not. It is clear that the condition is strongly affected by hormones, and hormone therapy is the favored treatment. I'd suggest minimizing your intake of estrogen from outside sources, such as commercially raised animal foods. Eat soy foods such as tofu, tempeh, and miso, which are rich in plant estrogens that can block more harmful forms of estrogen. Reduce the fat in your diet. Limit your alcohol intake. Make sure you get nourishing food and eat lots of fiber. Exercise regularly. Also, cut dairy foods from your diet. Try all this for one month and see whether it reduces the pain.

Stress will worsen this condition. Visualization, hypnotherapy, and Chinese medicine can all be helpful. You may want to consult with an herbalist as well. Dr. Christiane Northrup has an excellent chapter on endometriosis in *Women's Bodies, Women's Wisdom.* She suggests taking a multivitamin with plenty of B-complex and magnesium (about 50 milligrams of each of the B vitamins and 400 to 800 milligrams of magnesium), in addition to maintaining a low-fat, high-fiber diet.

Help for Halitosis?

Q:

I'm concerned about the causes and natural remedies for bad breath.

A:

The usual cause of bad breath is bacteria growing on the tongue, and sometimes around the gum line, too. There are a couple of simple ways to take care of the problem. First, try a tongue scraper. This is a metal instrument that you use to scrape your tongue once or twice a day, cleaning off bacteria. Second, you can brush your tongue with a germicidal toothpaste when you're brushing your teeth. Just take an extra thirty seconds to brush your tongue after you're done with your teeth, and try to include the back of your tongue—which will take some practice.

One product that works well is chlorine dioxide, which is in some regular toothpastes (for instance, Oxyfresh). Or go to a health food store and look for a toothpaste containing tea tree oil, an extract from the leaves of *Melaleuca alternifolia*, an Australian tree. Tea tree oil is a safe, powerful disinfectant that smells a bit like eucalyptus.

For temporary breath problems—say, when you return to work after a garlic-and-onion-laden lunch—try chewing on a bit of parsley or some fennel seeds. These will freshen your breath and also offer a nice finish to a meal. Try to stay away from products like Certs and Breath-Savers; they contain aspartame.

Bad breath is sometimes associated with gum disease. Check your gums for signs of irritation or swelling. If you notice a problem, talk to your dentist about it (he or she may refer you to a periodontist). Constant bad breath also may be a sign of systemic illness, especially liver disease or kidney disease. If it's a systemic problem, the breath is likely to have a distinct smell. Liver problems produce a mousy odor; severe bronchial infections will smell rotten. Sinusitis and inflammation inside the nose can also cause bad breath.

I wouldn't pay much attention to the claims made about mouthwashes like Scope or Listerine. These germicidal formulas may help, but they often don't penetrate into the crevices of the tongue. That's why I prefer brushing the tongue.

What to Do for Cracked, Dry Heels?

Q:

I have dry, cracked skin on my heels. I eat a healthy vegetarian diet and I scrub my heels with pumice to exfoliate the dead skin. Are the cracks a symptom of something else? Can you suggest a remedy?

A:

Problem dry heels are just that: dry heels. They're a common occurrence, especially in dry climates, and may show up seasonally. I have a big problem with them here in the desert because the heel cracks can become very painful if dirt gets in them or if they become deep.

Typically, if you wear socks, you'll regain the moisture on your heels and the cracks will go away. But I like to go barefoot or wear sandals. So it's an ongoing battle.

The key consideration for problem dry heels is finding a way to keep the cracks clean. The first thing I've found that really works to repair them is instant acrylic glue. It may sound crazy, but you just put a drop or two in the cleaned crack and press the edges together. The glue seals the skin and allows the healing to take place very quickly, often overnight. This also works for cracked fingertips.

Another possibility is to go to a pedicurist and get some professional loving-kindness directed at your feet. You can get footbaths, have the dead skin scraped off, and even get your toenails painted, if you like that kind of thing.

You may also want to try adding as much moisture as you can to your heels and feet. Water alone will extract moisture when it evaporates from your skin; oil protects, but can't add moisture. So the best moisturizer combines both.

Anything that stimulates circulation is also helpful: for example, a steam sauna with a cool water rinse between spells of heat.

Help for Hemorrhoids?

Q:

Being one of the masses who have desk jobs and take numerous plane trips, I often have hemorrhoids. Can you suggest any alternatives to the standard over-the-counter remedies?

A:

Hemorrhoids are distended veins around the anus that can become inflamed, causing itching, pain, and bleeding. They're not unusual at all; in fact, most people are bothered by them at some time or other. The pain can become severe. Prolonged sitting, constipation, and irritants in the diet are common causes. So is pregnancy. Stress can also make hemorrhoids flare up. Dietary irritants include strong spices such as red pepper and mustard, and drinks such as coffee, decaffeinated coffee, and alcohol. Avoid these, and tobacco.

You can treat constipation by eating more fiber. A vegetarian diet will help you here. Or take psyllium seed husks, in any of the forms available in drugstores and health food stores. Triphala, an herbal mixture from the Ayurvedic tradition, is an excellent bowel regulator. You can buy it in capsules in health food stores. Follow the dosage on the label. Drink lots of water—more than you think you need.

A natural, soothing treatment for the hemorrhoids themselves is an old-fashioned sitz bath. Sit in a bathtub filled with enough warm water to cover the anal area for fifteen minutes several times a day. Also, apply aloe vera gel to the area frequently. Instead of dry toilet paper, which will irritate the veins, use compresses of witch hazel to clean the anal area after bowel movements. You can buy witch hazel at any drugstore. Just moisten sheets of toilet paper with it. There are also pre-moistened, pre-packaged versions available.

Finally, here are two Chinese remedies that use foods to correct the imbalances that may cause hemorrhoids: Eat an orange three times a day, or eat two bananas first thing in the morning.

Healing Remedies for Herpes?

Q:

What do you recommend for treating genital herpes? I've tried acyclovir, and I've found it interrupts the virus's behavior but does nothing for healing the body. I've also been taking L-lysine three times a day and have found this to be effective. While I'm at it: Any thoughts about treating herpes on the lips?

A:

As you learned, acyclovir is less than ideal. It's expensive, may have side effects, and merely suppresses the symptoms without correcting the problem. L-lysine, an amino acid present in various foods, is worth trying because it inhibits replication of the herpes virus. I recommend 500 to 1,000 milligrams a day on an empty stomach. You can enhance L-lysine's effectiveness by minimizing foods like nuts, seeds, peas, and chocolate. In my experience, L-lysine is more effective with oral herpes than genital.

You might want to experiment with another natural

product: red marine algae (of the family *Dumontiaceae*), marketed under the name Intracept Pro (made by In Life Energy Systems). In lab tests, red marine algae appears to inhibit the herpes virus, although definitive human tests are lacking.

Many people have seen their herpes go into complete remission as a result of changes in lifestyle and mental attitude. Others have experienced significantly fewer flare-ups after trying visualizations and mental affirmations that tell the virus it's welcome in the body as long as it stays in the dormant stage. There's definitely the possibility of living in balance with the organism even if you can't get rid of it.

Got the Hiccups?

Q:

How best to get rid of hiccups?

A:

Hiccups are spasms of the diaphragm, followed by sudden closure of the glottis (the opening between the vocal cords), which temporarily stops the inflow of air. They can result from stress, excitement, stomach irritation, toxins, temperature changes, and other triggers. The root cause is irritability of the phrenic nerves along the spinal column; these nerves control the diaphragm.

Sometimes hiccups go away within a few minutes, and sometimes they last a long time. The longest-term sufferer known was an American pig farmer who hiccuped from 1922 to 1987.

Hiccups often resist the most ingenious treatment methods, so it's good to have several options in mind. You can try standing on your head, or swallowing crushed ice or dry bread, or drinking a glass of water rapidly. Another remedy is to make ginger tea and add honey, then sip it for ten minutes. Some people swear by putting a teaspoon of sugar or honey on the back of the tongue and swallowing it slowly. One remedy I've never had a chance to try involves drinking from a glass of water with a spoon in it while touching the end of the spoon to one ear. Another is asking a good friend to shout "boo" unexpectedly and scare you into breathing evenly.

My favorite method is to breathe in and out of a paper bag held over the nose and the mouth. This raises the carbon dioxide level of the blood, calming the phrenic nerves and diaphragm. (Don't use a plastic bag, though, because it can cling to your nostrils.) Keep breathing into the paper bag until the hiccups stop, or you feel uncomfortable.

What's the Buzz on Hives?

Q:

I get hives when my body temperature rises. What is the cause of this? I break out in a rash and experience profound itching. Please help me!

A:

You have an instability of the histamine system. Histamine is a biological response modifier, which is released in inflammatory and allergic reactions. Hives are very common, with about 20 percent of people experiencing them at one time or another. You're a long way toward a solution by noticing what triggers the itchy, rash-like bumps. In some people, hives can be set off by stress; in others, by food sensitivities, and in still others by the kind of temperature changes you describe. Three-quarters of the time, the reaction disappears within about eight months. It almost always goes away within a couple of years.

Conventional medicine is not of great help here. I

would recommend that you try a course of quercetin. Quercetin is a bioflavonoid from buckwheat and citrus fruits. It works by stabilizing the membranes of cells that release histamine, bringing allergic reactions under control. You can buy quercetin products in health food stores. The best form is a coated 400-milligram tablet, taken twice a day between meals.

Cornstarch or colloidal oatmeal added to your bathwater can soothe the itching. Aveeno bath treatment, available at drugstores, is one good oatmeal product.

You may also want to include plenty of garlic and onions in your diet, since they decrease histamine production.

Keep in mind that emotional upsets and stress are a very important trigger of hives: there is a definite mind-body connection with the histamine system. I would recommend working with a hypnotherapist or practitioner of visualization therapy who can help you quiet the condition.

Help for Hot Flashes?

Q:

I have tried herb after herb and I still can't find the right combination to get rid of my hot flashes. I'm desperate. Can you help?

A:

It's interesting how medicine has transformed a natural phase in the cycle of women's bodies into a disorder. For many years, it was considered impolite even to mention the word (that's when menopause was referred to as "the change"). Then menopause became one in a long list of imbalances attributed to women's reproductive systems, with proper intervention mandated. Pharmaceutical companies and gynecologists bombard women with the same message: Menopause is a time of unhappiness, bringing moodiness, hot flashes, osteoporosis, and loss of youthful attractiveness. The "life change" is actually a deficiency disease, the theory goes, and so only estrogen replacement therapy can restore vibrancy to women's bodies.

I'd recommend looking at this time of life in a new way. Instead of signifying aging and the loss of child-bearing ability, menopause can be a time to discover new energy, a freer self, and deeper wisdom within. Yes, there are discomforts associated with the changes in your body during this time. But these are signs of an opportunity to discover and claim the power of the second half of life.

During menopause, your body is adjusting to a change in hormone production. The ovaries stop releasing eggs, and it's no longer possible to get pregnant. The pituitary hormones, follicle-stimulating hormone (FSH), and luteinizing hormone (LH), which normally cycle during the month, begin to flow continuously at high levels. The ovaries slow down their output of estrogen, progesterone, and androgens. At the same time, other sites, such as the adrenal gland, the skin, and the brain, may take over hormone production. The ease of the transition depends greatly on a woman's stress level, emotional health, and nutritional status.

We rarely hear about women who have few problems with menopause, even though there are many of them. In non-Western cultures, menopause is often considered a time of strengthening and health for women. So first of all, it's important not to buy into the negative images and attitudes surrounding menopause in our culture.

Around 85 percent of American women experience the hot flashes you mention during menopause. Not long ago, Jane Fonda described her first hot flash this way: "When Ted and I were courting at a sound-and-light show in Athens, Greece, I had my first hot flash. It was dramatic and kind of exciting." You may feel a great heat around your head and neck, sweat profusely, then feel chilled. Some women go through these episodes for a few months, some for years. Hot flashes have been linked to blocked energy and unused sexual potential, so women who fear they will lose their sex drive with menopause may be more bothered by them. One tactic is to work to free your sexual energy and overcome the messages you are getting about an expected loss of sex drive.

I personally recommend a menopausal formula that works well for most women. Buy capsules or tinctures of these herbs at a health food store: dong quai, a female tonic made from the root of *Angelica sinensis*; vitex, or chaste tree (*Vitex agnus-castus*), a regulator of the female reproductive system; and damiana (*Turnera diffusa*), a plant that has a reputation as a tonic and female aphrodisiac. Take two capsules of each of these every day at noon, or one dropperful of each tincture mixed in warm water once a day at noon. Keep taking the herbs until you don't experience any hot flashes, then begin to reduce the dose and try to stop altogether.

Another herb widely used for menopausal discomforts, including hot flashes, is black cohosh (*Cimifuga racemosa*), now available in a commercial product called Remifemin. Its effectiveness is supported by good scientific data.

Many women also find ginseng to be very helpful for hot flashes, especially in combination with vitamin E (800 IU a day of the natural form). Nutrition is also important. Soy products contain estrogenlike substances that may account for the low incidence of menopausal symptoms in Japanese women. And researchers have found that deep, slow breathing can reduce hot flashes by half, probably by calming the central nervous system.

Finally, there are other Chinese herbs that help to relieve the problem; I'd suggest you visit a practitioner of traditional Chinese medicine if you want to learn about them.

How to Lick Lyme Disease?

Q:

We live in a wooded area in central Wisconsin and often have deer in our backyard. What is a safe way to protect our two-year-old son and ourselves from ticks? Are products like Deep Woods Off! safe for small children? Our son has already had two ticks on him this year. (I don't think they were deer ticks as they were pretty large.) Any info on ticks and Lyme disease would be appreciated.

A:

Lyme disease is an infection caused by an organism called *Borrelia burgdorferi*. It's named after Old Lyme, Connecticut, where doctors discovered the disease when they thought they were dealing with an epidemic of juvenile rheumatoid arthritis. There were about 8,000 cases of it in the United States in 1993, the most recent year for which I have figures.

Lyme disease presents a curious situation. There's a tremendous fascination with it as an exotic illness. And people are fearful of it because the symptoms can persist years after infection, even with treatment. So there's a tendency to rush to this diagnosis whenever patients have strange, persistent symptoms.

At the same time, a definitive diagnosis is often missed. Some physicians don't think to look for it and thus fail to give the proper treatment. To further complicate matters, we don't have a conclusive test for Lyme disease and there's no way of being sure it is the cause of any specific symptom.

Lyme disease is usually treated with up to one month of antibiotics. If these are administered at the right time in the right way, they should eradicate the organism.

If the disease is left untreated, about two-thirds of people infected develop recurring bouts of arthritis—sometimes years after the initial infection. The disease has also been associated with neurological symptoms, although it's not clear how severe they may be.

As you say, deer ticks host the organism. Deer, deer mice, and field mice carry the ticks, which are so small, they're practically invisible until fully engorged with blood—and then they are still hard to see. So the ticks you saw were not deer ticks. You should find out whether deer ticks are present in your area, and if so, whether they carry the bacteria that causes Lyme disease.

Generally I don't recommend any chemical pesticides. The only safe insecticide is pyrethrum, which is made from the flowers of certain chrysanthemum relatives. In areas where the disease is really prevalent, like Long Island and Connecticut, the best prevention is to wear protective clothing when you go out into the woods. Wear light colors and long sleeves, and tuck your pants into your socks. When you get back, wash immediately and keep an eye out for anything unusual on your body.

If you do have any odd symptoms like strange skin rashes, fever, or joint pain, go to a doctor who is knowledgeable about diagnosing and treating Lyme disease. The typical presentation is a rash in concentric rings, like a bull's-eye. But in many cases the rash is not present.

Help for Migraines?

Q:

What is the best natural cure for migraine headaches?

A:

Migraines are very unpleasant, often putting people out of action for days at a time as well as frustrating doctors, who frequently find that their arsenal of medications doesn't do the job.

Allergy, hormonal fluctuations, stress, and heredity are all factors that trigger attacks. My recommendations include:

- Eliminate coffee and decaf (and other sources of caffeine). Once a patient is off caffeine, coffee can be used as a treatment. Drink one or two cups of strong coffee at the first sign of an attack, then go lie down in a dark room.
- Eliminate other dietary triggers like chocolate, red wine (sometimes white wine, too), strong-flavored cheeses,

fermented foods (like soy sauce and miso), sardines, anchovies, and pickled herring.

- As a preventive, take feverfew herb (*Tanacetum parthenium*), a little plant related to chrysanthemum. You can buy a plant at a local nursery—it's a common ornamental—and chew a few leaves a day (be warned: they don't taste great), or you can buy a standardized extract at any health food store. Read the label to make sure it has the necessary active components, parthenolides, in it. One or two tablets or capsules a day will significantly reduce the frequency of migraines in many people. You can stay on feverfew indefinitely.
- Take a course of biofeedback training and learn how to raise the temperature of your hands. This will be a helpful tool to abort a headache at the start of an attack. To find a practitioner near you, look in the yellow pages or contact the Biofeedback Certification Institute of America.
- Use prescription medications sparingly. Try ergotamine to abort migraine attacks; it is a powerful constrictor of arteries that in order to work must be used at the first sign of an attack.
- Don't take Fiorinal on a regular basis. Many doctors prescribe it like candy to migraine sufferers without telling them that it contains an addictive downer (butalbital) and caffeine, as well as aspirin. Don't take prednisone or other steroids to prevent attacks; the potential dangers outweigh the benefits.

If you continue to have attacks, consider changing the way you think about your headaches. Migraine is like an electrical storm in the brain—violent and disruptive—but leading to a calm, clear state in the end. It's not so bad to have a headache once in a while; it actually can be a good excuse to drop routines, focus inwardly, and let stress dissipate. If you can come to accept the attacks in this way, they may occur less frequently.

Knocked Out by Narcolepsy?

Q:

I was diagnosed with narcolepsy in 1989. However, the medication that I take—Dexedrine 5-milligram tablets two to four times a day—does not seem to be working as it once did. I take medication vacations on the weekends thinking that I will regain the same action that it once gave me. Are there any new meds on the market or alternative methods that you can suggest?

A:

Narcolepsy can be disabling. A neurological disorder, it makes people excessively sleepy at unpredictable times. People who have it may find it unbearably hard to stay awake during meetings or music recitals, while driving, during a conversation, whenever. Then, at night, it may be difficult to get restful sleep, in part because of vivid dreams.

You didn't mention the other condition that is linked with narcolepsy, called cataplexy, a sudden loss of voluntary muscle control without warning, usually triggered by strong emotion. People with cataplexy suddenly fall to the ground when anything makes them laugh or cry. Physical exercise, too, can cause the reaction, which usually lasts for just a few seconds.

About 1 in 2,000 people has narcolepsy. Lots of times it's not diagnosed because people ignore their chronic sleepiness. There are also mild forms of cataplexy that cause people to drop objects or sit down suddenly.

The root cause of narcolepsy remains a mystery to neurologists. At Stanford University, researchers are studying a colony of Doberman pinschers, Labrador retrievers, and mixed breeds that have inherited the condition. They have linked the condition in dogs to a single gene that looks a lot like one of the human genes involved in managing the immune system. In humans, researchers found a gene called HLA-DR2 or HLA-DQwl in 98 percent of people with narcolepsy, but one-quarter of people without the condition also had HLA-DQwl, so there must be something else going on.

A neuroscientist at the University of California in Los Angeles has pinpointed a group of neurons that seem to fire at the wrong times, causing a mixup of waking and sleeping states. People with narcolepsy can go on dreaming while they're awake, and when they're asleep, their brains may be operating as if they were awake. Some scientists think that cataplexy may happen when a person shifts into the paralysis of REM sleep during waking hours.

Doctors tend to prescribe tricyclic antidepressants like

imipramine (Tofranil) or protriptyline (Vivactil) for cataplexy. They usually rely on stimulants to treat narcolepsy. But these can have significant side effects, such as anxiety, dependence, euphoria—and the one you describe, tolerance over time. Dexedrine is an old treatment and probably not the best choice anymore.

A company called Cephalon is planning to file for regulatory approval to sell one new drug, called modafinil (Provigil), this year. It's supposed to provide a substantial decrease in sleepiness with only minor side effects. Another possibility is yohimbine, from the bark of a West African tree, *Pausinystalia yohimbe*. In a small 1994 test, seven of eight men who took yohimbine were able to stay alert all day. One drawback is, again, the possibility of building tolerance. And some people have problems with stomach upset and flushing. But you might want to check with your doctor before taking either of these drugs.

As for nondrug treatments, it would be interesting to look at brain wave biofeedback. People can learn to condition fast-alert waves when they start to feel sleepy.

Some people also find several short catnaps (fifteen to twenty minutes) throughout the day to be a good coping strategy.

The National Sleep Foundation, at (202) 785-2300, is collecting a database of people with narcolepsy, their family histories, and biological samples. They hope to connect patients with researchers for clinical studies. There is also a patient support group called the Narcolepsy Network.

Pained by Plantar Warts?

Q:

My nine-year-old daughter has a few hard, white spots on the soles of her feet. I thought they might be plantar warts, as she goes barefoot in her weekly karate classes, but I'm not sure. How can I tell? Is there anything else that could be causing these white spots? There are three small spots, on one foot only.

A:

Plantar warts are just warts on the bottom of the foot, which is called the plantar surface. Ta-da: plantar warts! And because you put the whole weight of your body on your feet every day, they often get inflamed and painful. Warts are caused by the human papillomavirus (HPV).

I'd guess your diagnosis is correct, but you can be sure by taking a closer look. Get a magnifying glass and see if these dots show the characteristic appearance of a wart, that is, not smooth and hard, but with a rough, corrugated surface. Usually there will be a soft center, with rough rings around it. You may also see little black dots in the warts, which are bits of coagulated blood. If the spots don't look like this, or grow progressively larger and more tender, your daughter could have foreign bodies, like splinters, lodged under her skin. Doctors put acid on warts, freeze them off, or use an electric spark to burn them. Earl Mindell, in his *Vitamin Bible*, suggests applying 28,000 IU of vitamin E (from oil-base capsules) externally, one to two times a day, plus 400 IU (dry form) taken internally three times a day. But the best approach, especially in young people, is healing by suggestion. That would be my treatment of choice.

Children are especially good at visualizing warts away. You can go to a hypnotherapist or guided imagery therapist for help, but I'd give it a try on my own first. Work with your daughter to come up with an image that has an emotional charge for her. And encourage her to use it at least twice a day, especially on going to bed and on waking. One man I know got rid of a troublesome wart by imagining a steam shovel scraping away at it morning and night. Maybe your daughter will want to imagine applying some of her martial arts techniques against the intruder. Working with mental imagery is a good way to mobilize your body's healing powers.

How to Soothe the Poison Ivy Itch?

Q:

What is the best way to cure or alleviate the itchiness of poison ivy or poison oak?

A:

About half the population is susceptible to poison ivy, poison oak, and poison sumac, all members of the genus *Rhus*. The itching, blistering reaction you get from these plants is caused by a T-cell response to urushiol, the allergenic component of the oil the plants produce. If you think you're one of the lucky ones who happen to be immune, beware: allergy to these plants can come and go quite suddenly.

The reaction usually occurs thirty-six to forty-eight hours after contact and lasts for about two weeks. You won't spread the rash by scratching the blisters, but it can spread internally around the body and surface in unexpected places.

Of course, the best defense against this family of

plants is to learn how to recognize its members and avoid them. They can grow as shrubs or vines, and can be spotted by their characteristic clusters of three leaflets. The leaves can be shiny green, red-green, or red, depending on the season. If you do touch one of the plants, wash the oil off with soap and water within twenty to thirty minutes of contact. After that, the oil soaks into the skin. Watch and wash your pets, too. One common way to get the rash is to touch a dog that has rubbed against a plant and picked up oil on its coat.

Tecnu sells a very effective over-the-counter product that will remove the oils of poison oak, ivy, or sumac from the skin up to twenty-four hours after contact. The company also makes a protective lotion that you can put on your skin before you go out in the woods. These are the best preventive products I've found.

The absolute best treatment I know for poison ivy is to get in the shower and run hot water—as hot as you can stand—over the affected area for five to ten minutes. This seems counterintuitive, because it will increase the itching. But after a few minutes, the nervous circuits seem to get overloaded and the itching stops for a long time. If you conscientiously repeat the hot water treatment whenever the itching returns, the whole reaction completes its cycle rapidly and your skin will return to normal.

While hot water works better than anything, you also can use calamine lotion as a topical treatment if you wish. I strongly recommend against taking oral prednisone or other steroids unless there are very severe symptoms, such as fever or difficulty in urinating. Don't use topical steroids, either. Steroids are toxic drugs that should be saved for serious conditions, not minor ones, since they suppress the immune system.

Ouch! Relief for a Sprain?

Q:

I sprained my ankle four weeks ago. The swelling shrank considerably at first, but has remained on a plateau for the past three weeks and does not appear to be getting any better. What can I do for it? Do bad sprains normally take a long time to heal?

A:

The swelling of sprains should go down fairly quickly. If it doesn't, there may be some reason why the fluid is obstructed.

I have two suggestions. First, try acupuncture treatment. I have found acupuncture to work very effectively, especially for swollen knees; it reduces pain and speeds healing.

Second, take supplements of bromelain; you can buy it in capsules from health food stores. This is a pineapple enzyme that's used by some sports doctors. I've seen it dramatically reduce swelling from injuries. The dose is

200 to 400 milligrams, three times a day. Take it between meals, on an empty stomach—at least ninety minutes before or three hours after eating. (Some people are allergic to bromelain, so stop using it if you develop any itching.)

The best way to reduce swelling and blood flow during the first twenty-four hours after a sprain is to put ice on it right away. You can buy wraparound ice packs or just use a bag of frozen peas or some ice cubes in a towel. Try to keep the ice on as much as possible for the first few hours; after that, intermittent applications may be helpful. After twenty-four hours, you can start alternating heat and cold. Protect the sprain from further injury by using a wraparound bandage.

Either tincture of arnica or DMSO (dimethyl sulfoxide) may ease the pain and swelling. Arnica is a plant native to the high mountains of western North America that can be crushed whole and soaked in alcohol to produce a soothing liniment. Rub it in gently, but not into broken skin. Never ingest tincture of arnica; it's toxic. But you can take homeopathic arnica tablets in the 30x potency. Start with four tablets as soon as possible after the injury, then take four more every hour for the first day. Place the tablets under your tongue and let them dissolve. The next day, take four tablets every two hours. Then, the following day, cut back to four tablets four times a day. You may continue this for four or five days.

DMSO is a chemical made from wood pulp. It penetrates the skin and promotes healing. Paint a 70 percent solution of DMSO on the sore area with cotton and let it dry. You may feel warmth or stinging, and experience a garlicky taste in your mouth. Try it three times a day for three days. If there is no improvement, stop using it. If you do feel some improvement, apply DMSO twice a day for three more days, then once a day for a final three days.

Why the Stye?

Q:

I have been getting styes lately. Would you know what causes them? Is it a bacterial infection or lack of a nutrient?

A:

Styes are bacterial infections of the tear duct. The technical name is hordeolum, usually caused by staph. They can be quite painful and disfiguring, causing the area around the eye to redden and swell. Usually they go away on their own, with patience.

Styes on the outside of your eyelid eventually will rupture, discharge pus, then disappear. Inside your eyelid, the infection can be more severe. You can speed the resolution of the problem by applying hot compresses for ten minutes a couple of times a day. Topical antibiotics usually don't help much.

Recurrence is not unusual. But if you're getting these regularly it would be a good idea to look for an underlying cause, such as contact lenses or exposure to cigarette smoke. Styes are contagious and can be transmitted by finger contact. But most people don't get them because the immune system protects the eyes pretty well. Our tears contain antibodies that eliminate bacteria before they get a chance to settle in. Sometimes the appearance of a stye can indicate a temporary depression of immunity.

I don't know of any nutritional lack that would cause styes, but it might be worth trying a regimen of vitamin C. I'd suggest 3,000 to 6,000 milligrams of vitamin C a day, in three equal doses, to see if this reduces the frequency of the infections you're experiencing.

Need to Dry Out Swimmer's Ear?

Q:

What's the best medicine for swimmer's ear?

A:

The best way to treat "swimmer's ear," like just about anything, is to avoid getting it in the first place (use wax or silicone earplugs). But if it's too late for that, make a mixture of equal parts white vinegar and rubbing alcohol. Get in the habit of rinsing your ears out with this potion when you come out of a pool or the ocean. Then gently dry your ears with a cotton swab.

Other preventive measures include shaking your head when you get out of the pool to expel trapped water. You can also place the tip of some clean facial tissue, twisted into a point, into each ear for about ten seconds to soak up the moisture. Don't remove earwax from your ears (unless it's a problem), because it helps protect the ear canal.

Once you've got swimmer's ear, you're probably going

to have to treat it with an antibiotic solution like Neosporin, which comes in a form specifically for ears.

I have two favorite remedies for earaches: garlic oil and mullein oil. Warm either of these oils slightly, then use a dropper to put a few drops in the ear that is hurting. Plug it loosely with cotton. To make garlic oil, crush a few cloves into some olive oil and let it sit for a few days, then strain it. Some people put a small piece of peeled raw garlic directly into the ear—it eventually dissolves. You can find mullein oil in health food stores. It's made by steeping the flowers from mullein—*Verbascum thapsus,* a common roadside weed—in olive oil. Apply it the same way as the garlic oil. Try it, it really works.

Will the Ringing Ever Stop?

Q:

I'm a massage therapist. One of my clients has experienced ringing in his ears for months. The only treatment his doctors advise is to continue on steroids, even though there has not been noticeable improvement. I read in Spontaneous Healing *about a German physician who experienced great success with yoga and stress relief techniques. Can you recommend an alternative? Any herbs?*

A:

Tinnitus—ringing in the ears—was relatively rare when I was in medical school, but it's definitely not rare these days. It has become almost epidemic in the United States, and there's not really any clear understanding among medical doctors of its cause. It seems to affect people of all ages, and the medical treatments for it aren't very good. Some people think it's due to a viral infection, but that's just the ready Western answer to many medical riddles.

What you hear are noises that come from inside the body and won't go away. It feels as if there's no way to escape, which can be most annoying. The noises can make it hard to hear other people's voices, to concentrate, or to sleep through the night.

As I wrote in *Spontaneous Healing*, my German physician friend, Helmut Milz, M.D., of Marquartstein, Bavaria, works at a psychosomatic medical clinic and regards tinnitus as a stress-related condition. He believes that chronic muscle tension in the head and neck interferes with blood circulation to the inner ear. If he's right, then increased use of computers, television watching, and the general stress in our culture could explain why there is so much more tinnitus these days.

I would recommend two approaches. First, your client should do some kind of stress reduction technique aimed specifically at improving posture and relaxing muscles. I would recommend yoga, or bodywork such as the Alexander technique. I would also suggest acupuncture.

Second, I would use the herb ginkgo (*Ginkgo biloba*). Ginkgo is nontoxic and increases blood circulation in the head and neck. Many people report improvement with it. Your client would need to take it for at least two months before making a decision about its usefulness. The dose is two tablets of the standardized extract three times a day, with meals.

Check out Richard Hallam's book *Tinnitus: Dealing with the Ringing in Your Ears*, which is based on the philosophy that the best way to deal with ringing is to stop fighting it. Hallam, who is a psychologist, helps readers learn to tolerate the sounds until they stop being annoying and aren't particularly noticeable. Another good resource is the American Tinnitus Association in Portland, Oregon.

What the $#@%!?

Q:

Tourette's syndrome is a disorder hallmarked by involuntary motor and vocal tics. Any info on new findings about this disorder? Any suggestions on natural therapies to relieve the symptoms? Some say it is related to obsessive-compulsive disorder. Any thoughts on this?

A:

Since Tourette's syndrome has become better known, many people are delighted by the concept—especially the thought of being able to yell "fuck" in public and get away with it.

But, of course, it's not that simple. As you say, people who have the disease experience a variety of uncontrollable "tics" that can range from simple motions like blinking to complex activities like bending over and touching the ground. People may also grunt, clear their throats, or bark. Inappropriate swearing, making obscene gestures, and compulsive imitation of others can also occur in this neuropsychiatric disorder, but they are far less common. More common, and very disturbing to Touretters, are surges of uncontrollable rage and other strong emotions.

A French neurologist named Georges Gille de la Tourette first identified the syndrome in 1885 after observing several patients, including a French noblewoman, the Marquise de Dampierre, who would make sudden bizarre cries in the middle of polite conversation. Until a couple of decades ago it was considered a psychiatric disorder, mostly of boys, brought on by poor parenting skills.

Now there's considerable evidence for a genetic root, combined with prenatal environmental factors and birth complications. Children with Tourette's often were exposed before birth to high levels of tobacco smoke, coffee, or alcohol. It's estimated that more than 100,000 Americans have the syndrome, with only one out of every four male. The syndrome is less associated with uninhibited angry outbursts in women, so some people speculate that the quiet, odd actions of young girls and women with the condition often go unnoticed and undiagnosed.

There are strong links with obsessive-compulsive disorder (OCD)—and a number of other psychiatric problems. Touretters often show obsessive-compulsive behavior like washing their hands repeatedly, as well as attention-deficit hyperactivity disorder (ADHD), and anxiety.

In fact, these symptoms often cause far more distress to the person than does Tourette's syndrome itself. And they can be difficult to treat, because the stimulants given for ADHD, for example, tend to worsen the tics. But many Touretters don't take any medication at all. As they grow older, they become practiced and comfortable explaining their condition to others when the tics happen in public. And they learn to suppress them. Family counseling and therapy are good ways to help the whole family deal with the stigma of socially unacceptable—or at least unusual—behavior.

The tics get worse under stress, so there's an obvious place to begin to find natural solutions to the problem. Biofeedback, relaxation techniques, and exercise may help. And some people have used the surges of behavioral changes as a creative resource. In his book *The Man Who Mistook His Wife for a Hat*, Oliver Sacks writes about a surgeon with Tourette's who maintains an active practice and skillfully performs extremely complex operations. Some people think Mozart had Tourette's.

To learn more about the disease, I suggest reading *A Mind of Its Own: Tourette's Syndrome, a Story and a Guide*, by Ruth Dowling Bruun and Bertel Bruun. There's also a film, *Twitch and Shout,* by Laurel Chiton, which you can get through New Day Films in New Jersey. Other resources include the Tourette Syndrome Association in Bayside, New York.

Cranberries for Urinary Tract Infections?

Q:

What is the latest on cranberries and urinary tract infections? If cranberries do help, can one use cranberry supplements rather than juice for the same effect?

A:

Urinary tract infections occur when bacteria such as E. coli, which normally live in the bowel, make their way into the bladder and set up residence. Cranberry juice, long recommended as a folk remedy for the problem, has held up under scientific scrutiny. In a study published in the *Journal of the American Medical Association*, women who drank cranberry juice were 58 percent less likely to develop a urinary tract infection than those who drank a placebo (another red drink containing vitamin C). If they already had an infection, they were 27 percent less likely to have their infections continue if they drank cranberry juice. Advocates of cranberry juice treatment used to think it worked by acidifying the urine, making it less hospitable to bacteria. But now it appears that cranberries (and blueberries) contain a substance that disrupts the glue that bacteria use to adhere to tissue, making it harder for them to get established on the lining of the bladder.

I'm with you on skipping the juice. Cranberry juice—at least the ordinary variety—is full of sugar and water, with only some of the real stuff. The high sugar content may actually encourage the growth of bacteria and yeast.

So my preference is to drink unsweetened cranberry juice concentrate, which you can buy in a health food store, or to buy capsules of cranberry extract. The Eclectic Institute makes a freeze-dried product that's good. Take two capsules twice a day. Even if you're taking pharmaceutical drugs to treat the infection, I'd still take cranberry along with them.

Another herbal treatment for bladder infections is uva ursi, also known as bearberry (*Arctostaphylos uva-ursi*). This kills bacteria and reduces inflammation. But don't use it for more than a week, because it can irritate your kidneys and upset your stomach. Also, you must keep your urine alkaline in order for the uva ursi to work. That means eating lots of fruits and vegetables, especially potatoes. For a little extra antibacterial punch, eat garlic, nasturtium, parsley, and rose hips whenever you can.

You can also take some measures to help prevent a return of the infection. Avoid tight pants, synthetic underwear, and deodorant soaps, all of which can encourage bacteria. Also, many women get urinary tract infections shortly after a pelvic exam. Drinking a glass of water just before and after visiting your gynecologist seems to help protect against this problem.

Natural Help for Yeast Infections?

Q:

What do I do about recurring yeast infections? I've had them for over twenty years.

A:

Many women suffer from frequent vaginal yeast infections, which can indicate an underlying metabolic imbalance. It often helps if you change your diet to make your body a less appealing host for the organism. Your partner may want to do the same. (Studies suggest that treating the patient's sexual partner may stop recurrence.)

First, try reducing your sugar intake. High-sugar diets stimulate the growth of yeast. Also, add garlic to your diet. A clove once a day is a powerful natural medicine, with specific anti-yeast effects. (That's one segment from a bulb, not the whole thing!) Mash or chop it fine, mix it with food, and eat it with a meal. Or cut it into chunks and swallow the chunks like pills. Fresh garlic is much better than any garlic supplement. Chew a little parsley afterward if you're concerned about odor—but if you eat garlic regularly and have a good attitude about it, you won't smell of it. Try it, it really works.

Finally, take acidophilus culture. These bacteria are the ones that make milk sour. "Friendly" and natural to the intestinal tract, they may also out-compete yeast in the vaginal area and change the chemistry of the tissues to make them resistant to the fungi. You can buy acidophilus in health food stores, in capsules or in a milk or carrot-juice base. Check the expiration date to make sure the bacteria are viable. Take 1 tablespoon of the liquid culture or one to two of the dry capsules after meals, unless the label directs otherwise.

These changes to your diet may help reverse some of your underlying susceptibility to yeast infections. To treat the infections when they occur, try placing a capsule of acidophilus directly into your vagina once a day, or use a rubber bulb syringe to insert one tablespoon of liquid culture. Another possibility would be tea tree oil, a nontoxic treatment very useful for fungal infections. You can find it in health food or herb stores. Mix 1½ tablespoons of the oil in a cup of warm water and use it as a douche once a day. If you experience any irritation, however, discontinue its use.

Resources

Books by Andrew Weil, M.D.

8 Weeks to Optimum Health: A Proven Program for Taking Full Advantage of Your Body's Natural Healing Power. New York: Alfred A. Knopf, 1997.

Spontaneous Healing: How to Discover and Enhance Your Body's Natural Ability to Maintain and Heal Itself. New York: Ballantine Books, 1996.

Natural Health, Natural Medicine: A Comprehensive Manual for Wellness and Self-Care. Rev. ed. Boston: Houghton Mifflin, 1995.

Health and Healing: Understanding Conventional and Alternative Medicine. Rev. ed. Boston: Houghton Mifflin, 1995.

From Chocolate to Morphine: Everything You Need to Know About Mind-Altering Drugs, with Winifred Rosen. Rev. ed. Boston: Houghton Mifflin, 1993.

The Natural Mind: An Investigation of Drugs and the Higher Consciousness. Rev. ed. Boston: Houghton Mifflin, 1986.

The Marriage of the Sun and the Moon: A Quest for Unity in Consciousness. Boston: Houghton Mifflin, 1980.

Other Recommended Books

Bruun, Ruth Dowling, and Bertel Bruun. *A Mind of Its Own: Tourette's Syndrome, a Story and a Guide.* New York: Oxford University Press, 1994.

Hallam, Richard. *Tinnitus: Dealing with the Ringing in Your Ears.* London: Thorsons, 1993.

Lerner, Michael. *Choice in Healing: Integrating the Best of Conventional and Alternative Approaches to Cancer.* Cambridge: MIT Press, 1994.

Mindell, Earl. *Vitamin Bible.* Rev. ed. New York: Warner Books, 1991.

Northrup, Christiane, M.D. *Women's Bodies, Women's Wisdom: Creating Physical and Emotional Health and Healing.* New York: Bantam Books, 1995.

Sacks, Oliver. *The Man Who Mistook His Wife for a Hat.* New York: Summit Books, 1985.

Sarno, John, M.D. *Healing Back Pain: The Mind-Body Connection.* New York: Warner Books, 1991.

Other Resources

American Tinnitus Foundation
P.O. Box 5
Portland, OR 97207
503 248-9985

Biofeedback Certification Institute of America
10200 West 44th Avenue, Suite 304
Wheat Ridge, CO 80033
303 420-2902

Eclectic Institute
14385 Southeast Lusted Road
Sandy, OR 97055
503 668-4120 or 800 332-4372
Fax: 503 668-3227

In Life Energy Systems
107 California Avenue
Mill Valley, CA 94941
415 389-1738

National Sleep Foundation
1367 Connecticut Avenue NW, Suite 200
Washington, DC 20036
202 785-2300

New Day Films
201 652-6590

Tourette Syndrome Association
42-40 Bell Boulevard
Bayside, NY 11361
718 224-2999

Program in Integrative Medicine

At the University of Arizona Health Sciences Center, Tucson, Arizona. For more information, visit the Web site: http://www.ahsc.arizona.edu/integrative_medicine. Or write: Center for Integrative Medicine, P.O. Box 64089, Tucson, AZ 85718.

Newsletter

If you would like more information on my lectures and informational products, including my monthly newsletter, *Self Healing,* please write to: Andrew Weil, M.D., P.O. Box 457, Vail, AZ 85641.

On the Web

"Ask Dr. Weil" answers health questions daily on Time Warner's Pathfinder Network (www.drweil.com).

Index

About Andrew Weil, M.D.

Dr. Andrew Weil is the leader in the new field of Integrative Medicine, which combines the best ideas and practices of conventional and alternative medicine. A graduate of Harvard Medical School, he is director of the Program in Integrative Medicine at the University of Arizona, the first program to train physicians in this way at an American medical school. He is also the founder of the Center for Integrative Medicine in Tucson, which is advancing the field worldwide. Dr. Weil is well known as an expert in natural medicine, mind-body interactions, and medical botany, as well as the author of the bestselling *Spontaneous Healing* and *8 Weeks to Optimum Health*. According to Dr. Weil, "Spontaneous healing is not a miracle or a lucky exception, but a fact of biology, the result of the natural healing system that each of us is born with."

About "Ask Dr. Weil"

The "Ask Dr. Weil" program (www.drweil.com) features Andrew Weil, M.D., and is one of the top-rated health sites on the World Wide Web and is featured on Time Warner's Pathfinder Network. The recipient of many awards, the "Ask Dr. Weil" program features a daily

Q&A with answers to a wide range of health questions, a daily poll, and the Doc Weil Database, which lets readers search hundreds of topics, including material from Dr. Weil's bestselling book *Natural Health, Natural Medicine.* The site also features a Referral Directory (practitioners from acupuncture to Trager work) and DocTalk, a live weekly chat with Dr. Weil. If you have additional questions for Dr. Weil, ask them on his Web site.

About Steven Petrow (Series Editor)

Steven Petrow is the executive producer of the "Ask Dr. Weil" program. Mr. Petrow has held editorial positions with *Life* magazine, *Longevity* magazine, *Fitness*, and *The Wall Street Journal.* He's also been the editor-in-chief of *10 Percent* magazine and *AIDS Digest* and has published five books, including *The HIV Drug Book* and *When Someone You Know Has AIDS.*

Acknowledgments

Richard Pine, Judith Curr, Elisa Wares, and Scott Fagan

[illegible]

About Steven [illegible] (Series Editor)

[illegible]

Acknowledgments

[illegible]